# MY MOM IS A RESPIRATORY THERAPIST

By: Dr. Tabatha M. Dragonberry DHSc, MEd, MBA, RRT-NPS, RRT-ACCS, AE-C, CPFT, C-NPT

&

Phyllis A. Teeter

Illustrated by: Pixelgraphics

**DEDICATED TO ALL THE MOM RESPIRATORY THERAPISTS WHO WORK 365/24/7 CARING FOR OTHERS! WE APPRECIATE YOU!**

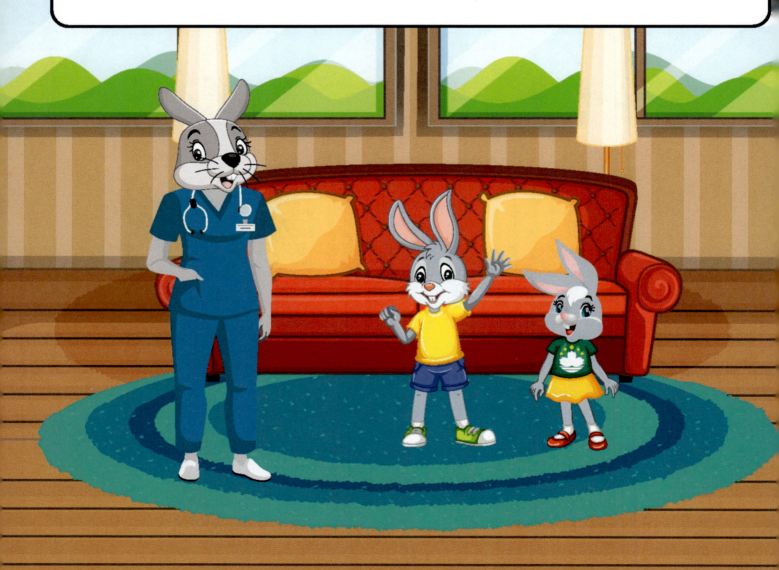

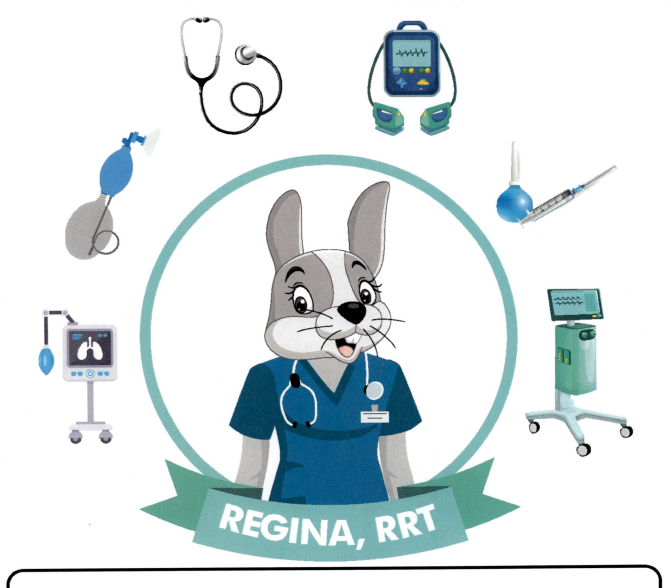

Regina Rabbit is her name and Respiratory care is her game.

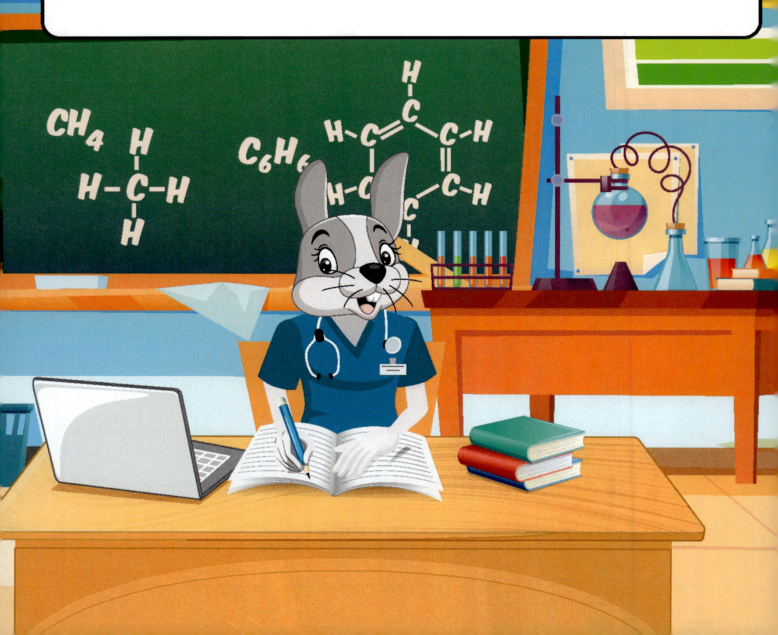

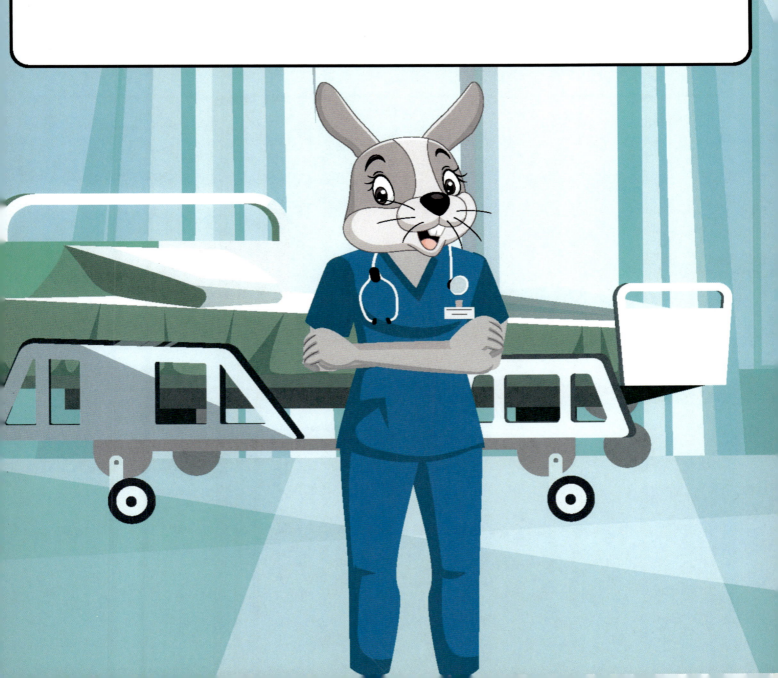

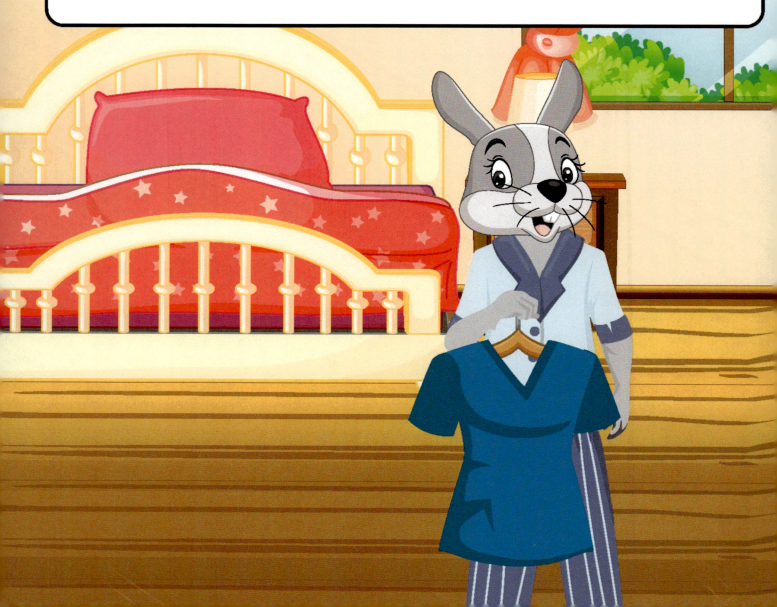

She gets up early as can be to take care of patients just like you and me.

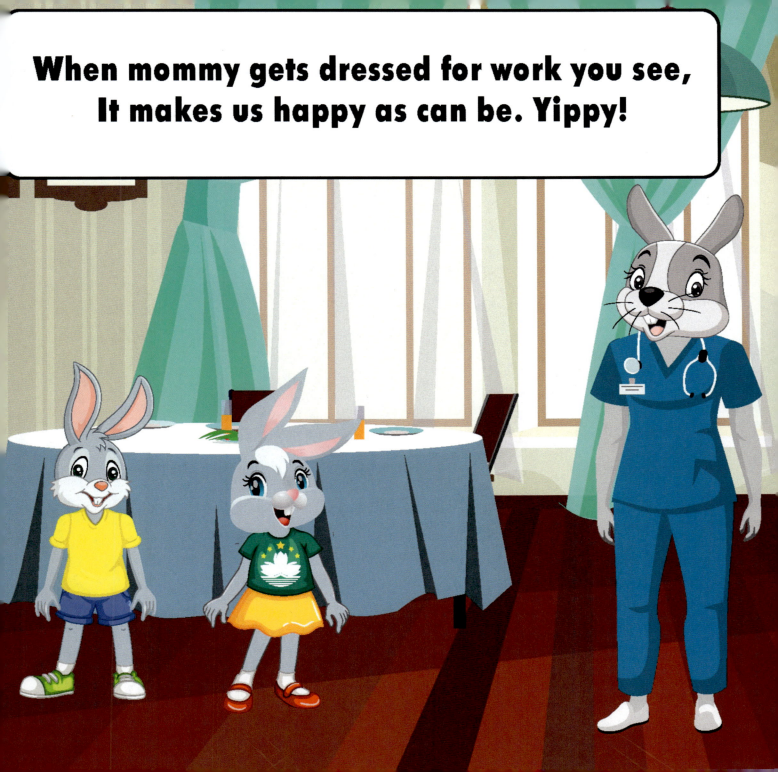

Her day starts out with a morning commute sometimes she gets stuck in traffic to boot.

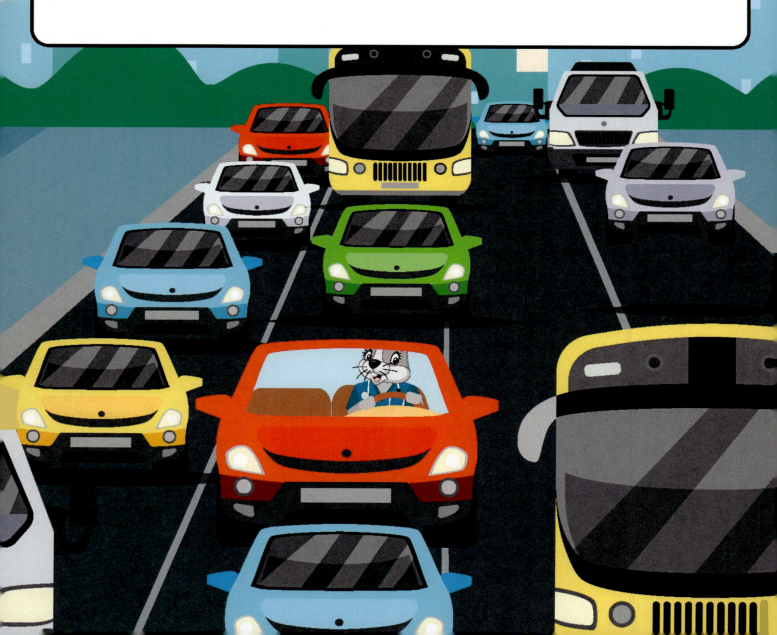

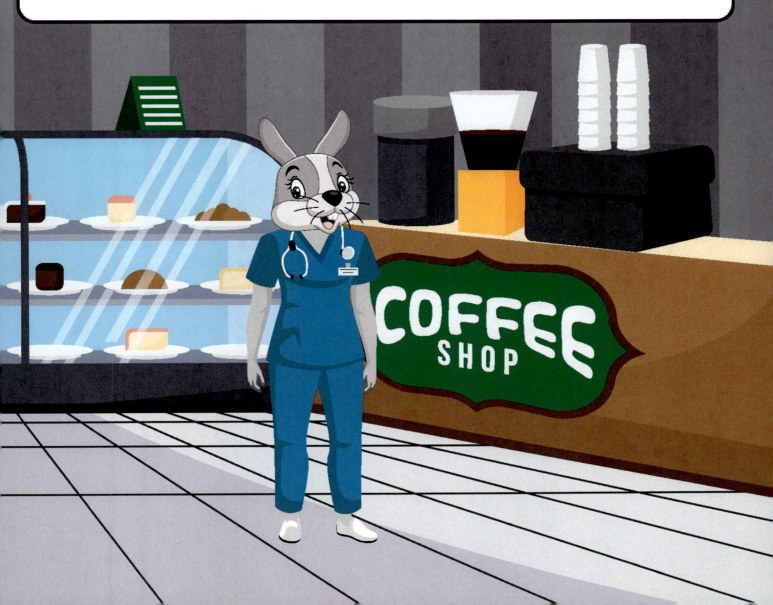

She stops for a coffee along the way to stop zombie mommy from going astray.

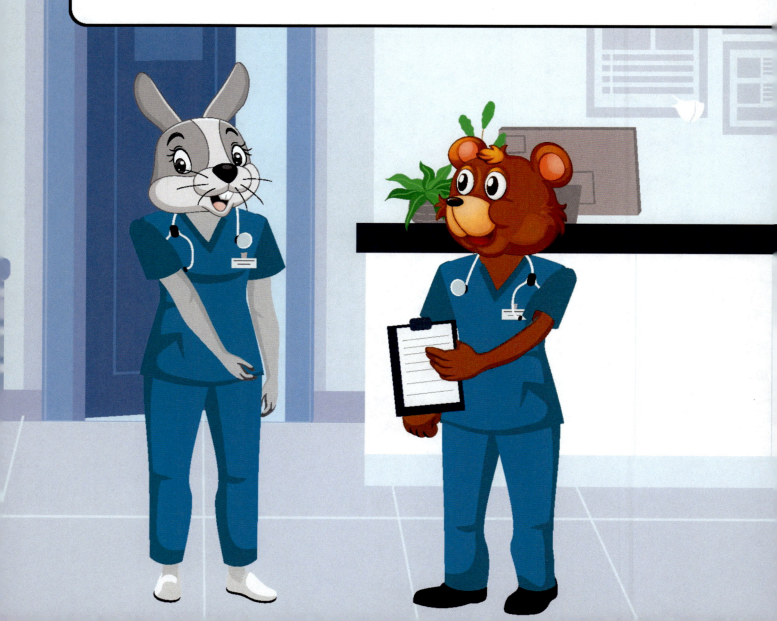

He cared for the patients the night before, and he is ready to walk out that door.

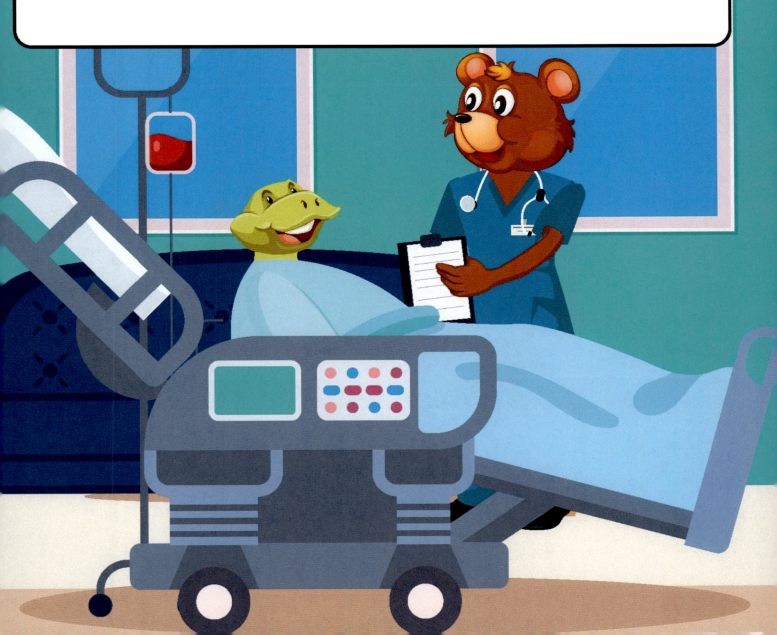

**Now! It's mommy's time to go to the floor. Her day is never a bore.**

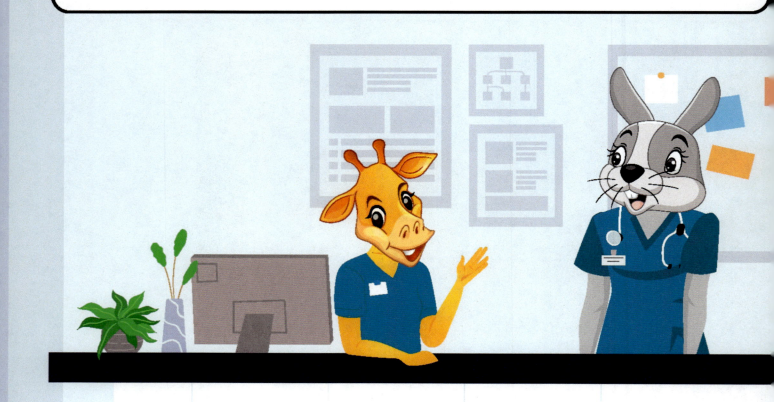

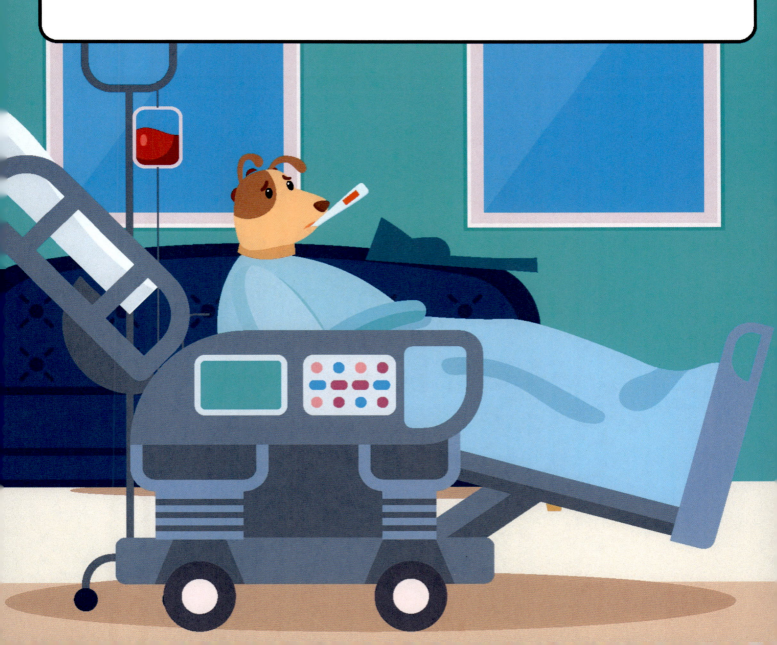

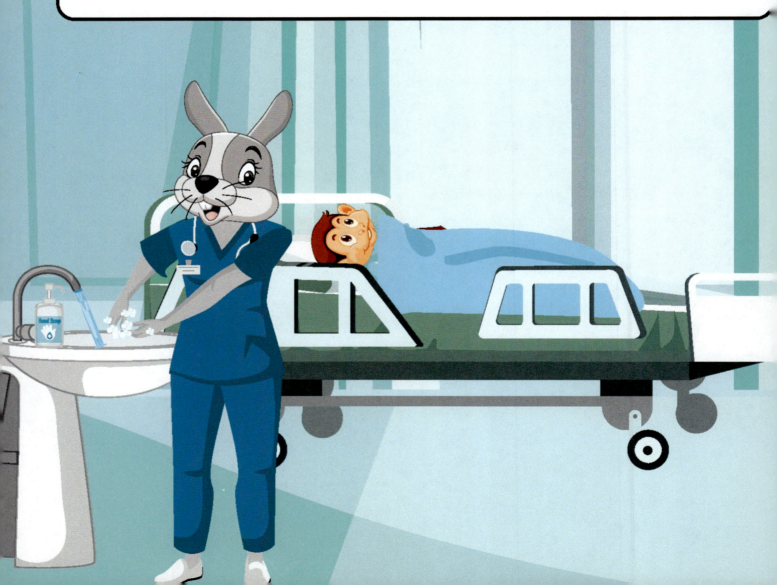

She washes her hands to be sure they're clean.
She can't pass out germs that would be mean.

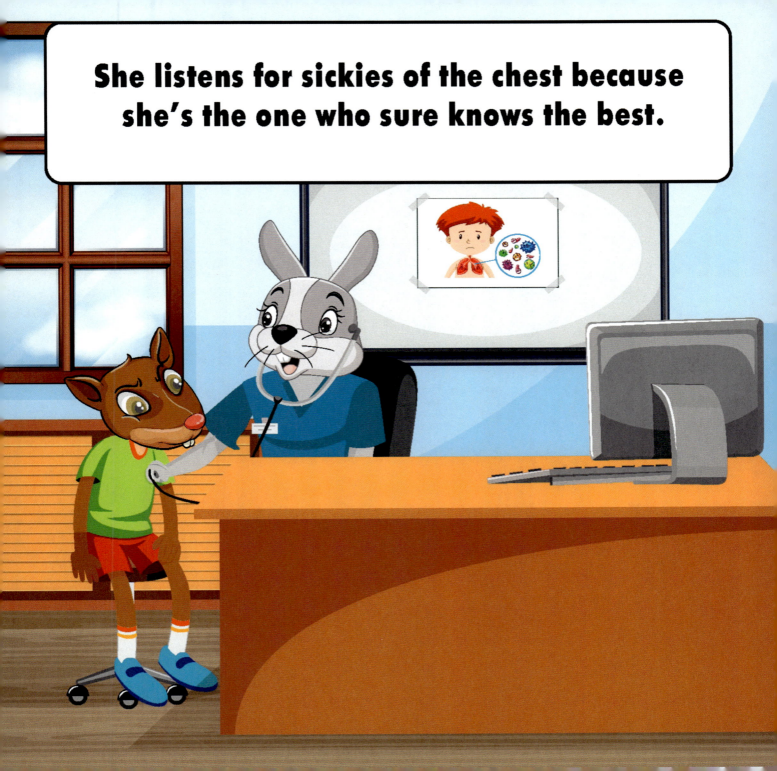

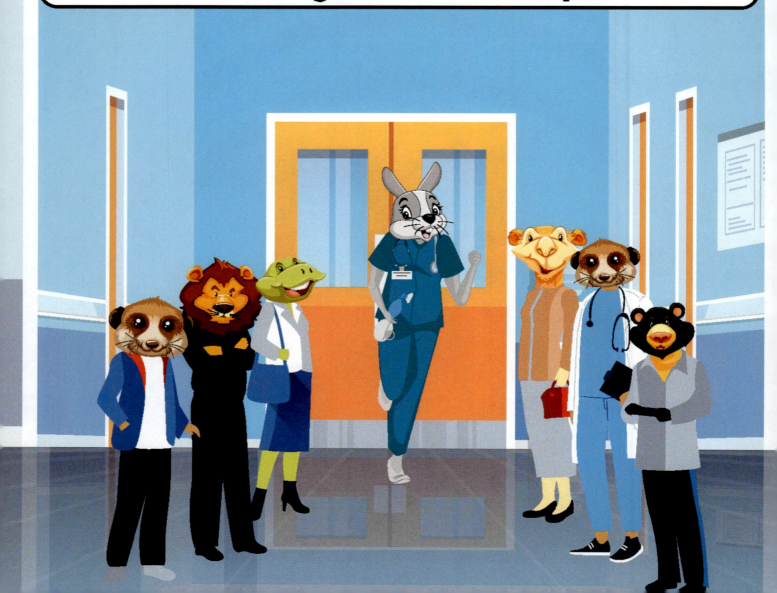

When she hears something bad, she won't even get mad. That means she is needed to save the day and everyone must get out of her way.

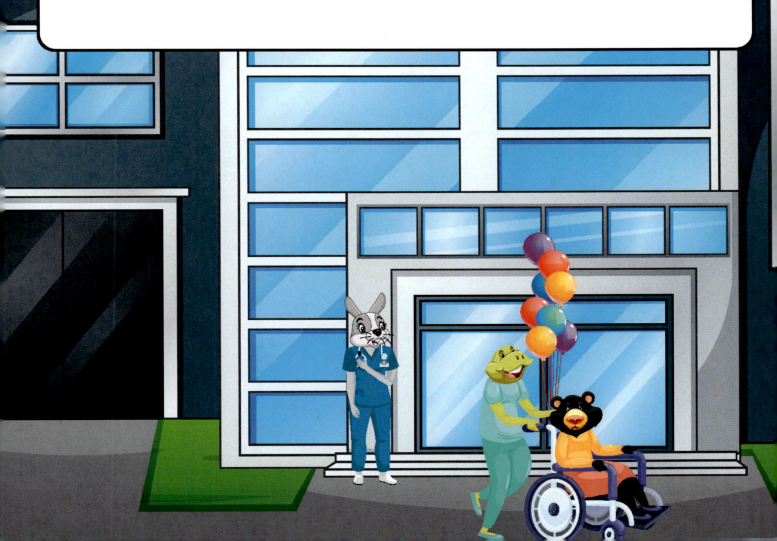

This warms her heart because she is doing her part.

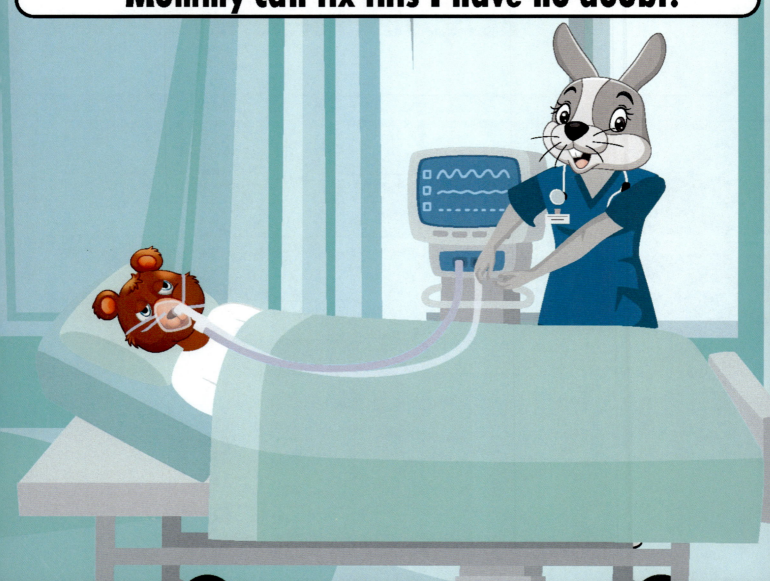

Some of the patients get pretty wheezy and this is when breathing ain't easy.
Squeaks on the way in and out.
Mommy can fix this I have no doubt.

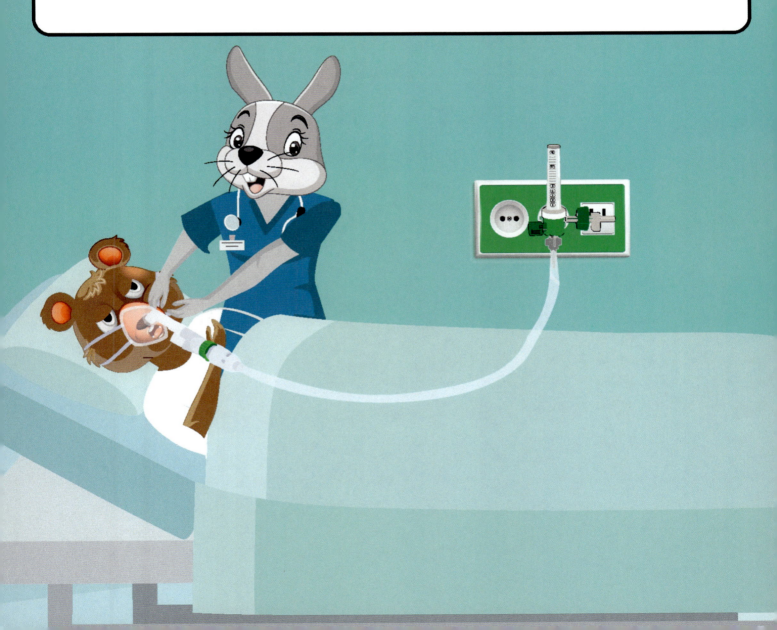

She mixes the medicine in a cup so patients can breathe it all up. The misty spray is even better than grandma's crochet.

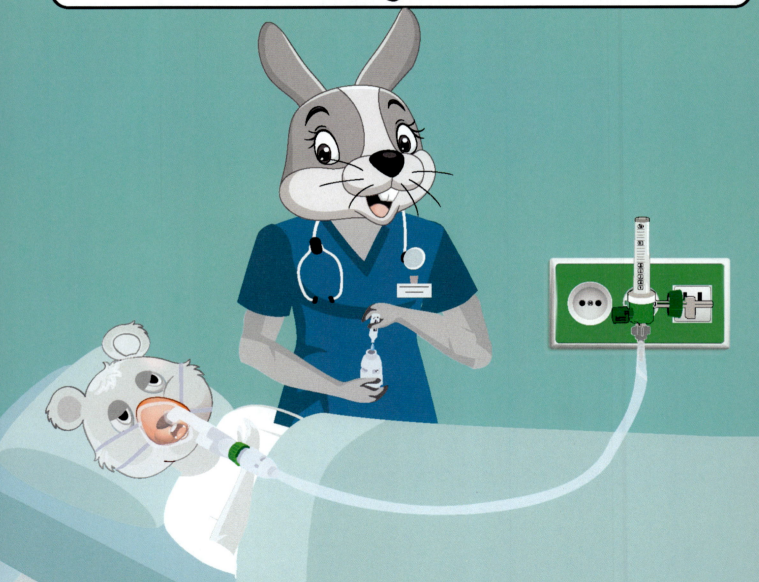

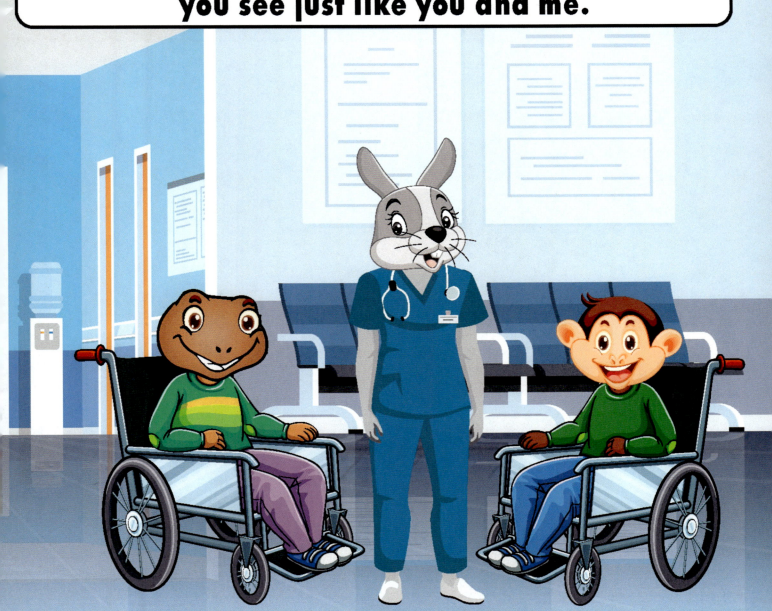

Albuterol is the medicine she picks. Oh! It sure does the trick. It makes the patients all better real quick. Albuterol is super special, you see just like you and me.

Clapping, cupping, and chest physio
knock the phlegm loose and give it a go.
Cough it up, cough it up, my friend.
My mom will clear those lungs up in the end.

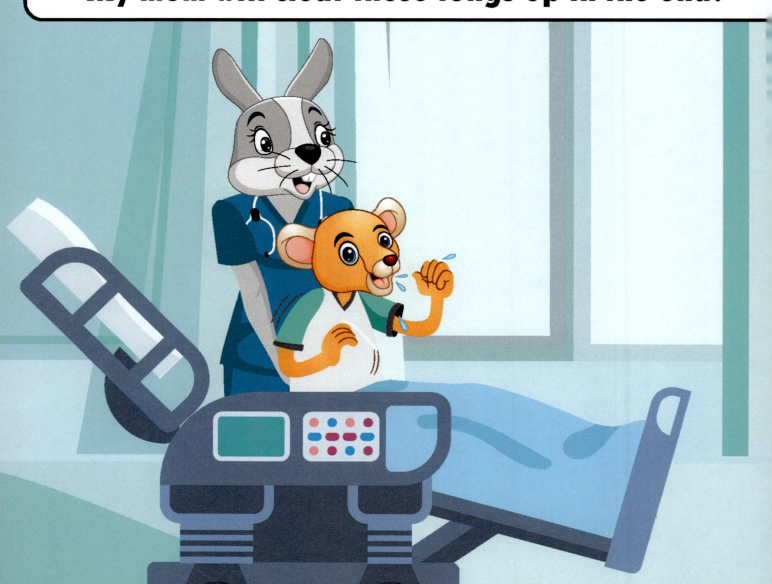

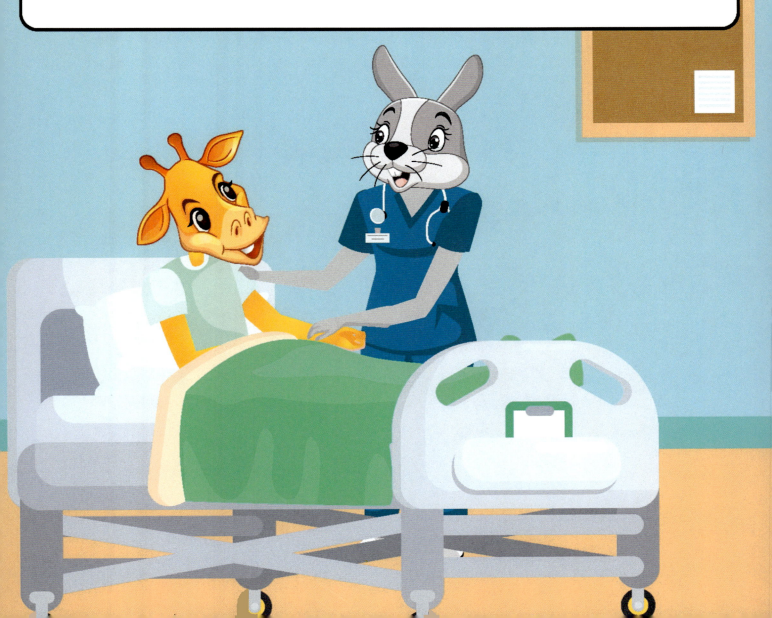

Keep calm you see because our mom is a super RT. No tears or fears, mommy helps them get better for years.

Over the loudspeaker, you can hear! Regina the Rabbit, RRT, you are needed as fast as can be!

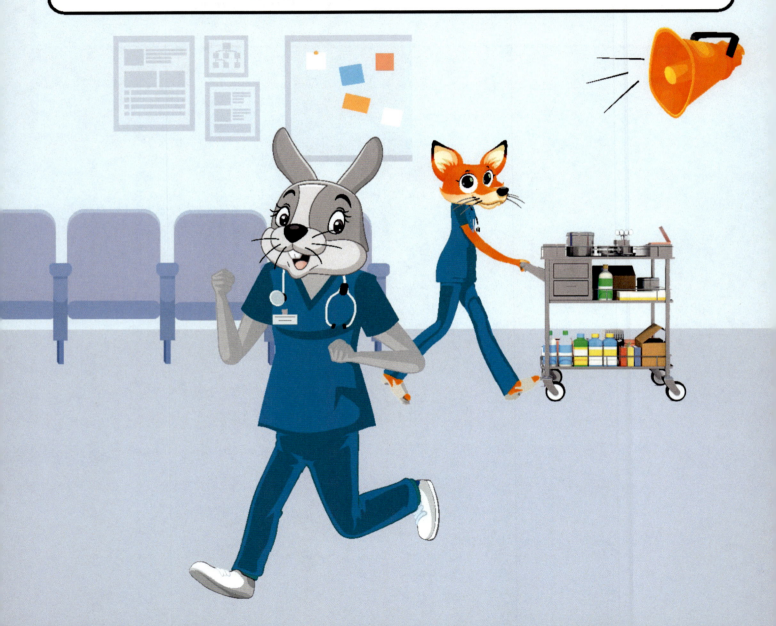

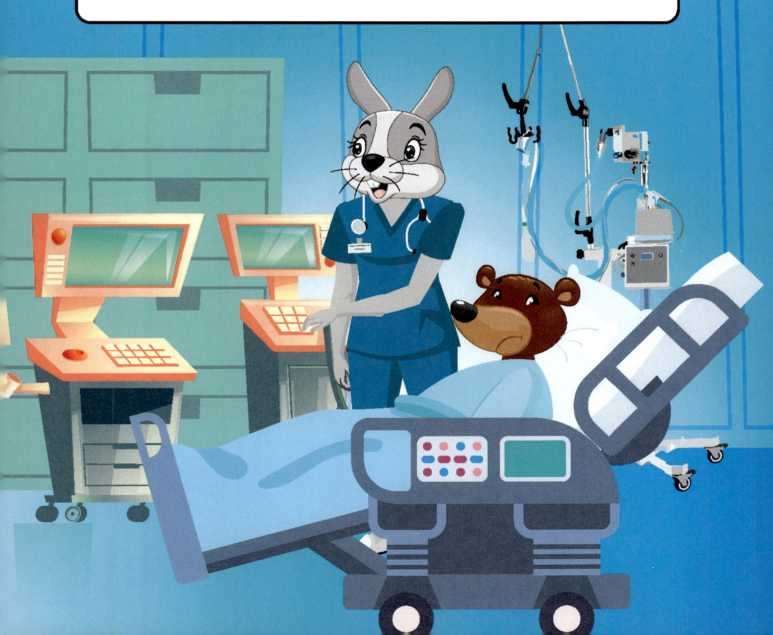

Sometimes she works in the ICU this is where she really knows what to do.
It's where the sickest of the sick do go.

With eyes like a hawk, she keeps watching every day to care for her patients in every way. The lungs are special and deep inside but do not do well when they are tried.

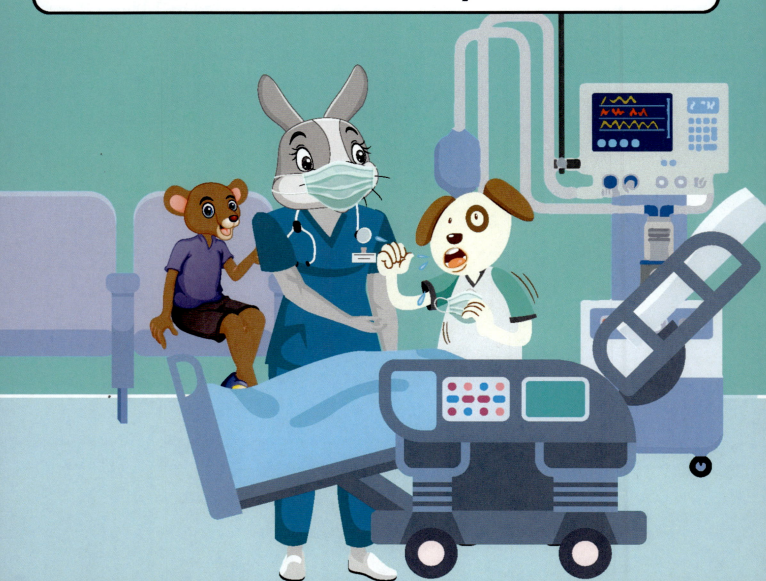

**Ventilators are her favorite tool. She controls the pressure because she's so cool. The Vent Swooshes air in and the air Swooshes out just to help the patient's lungs right out.**

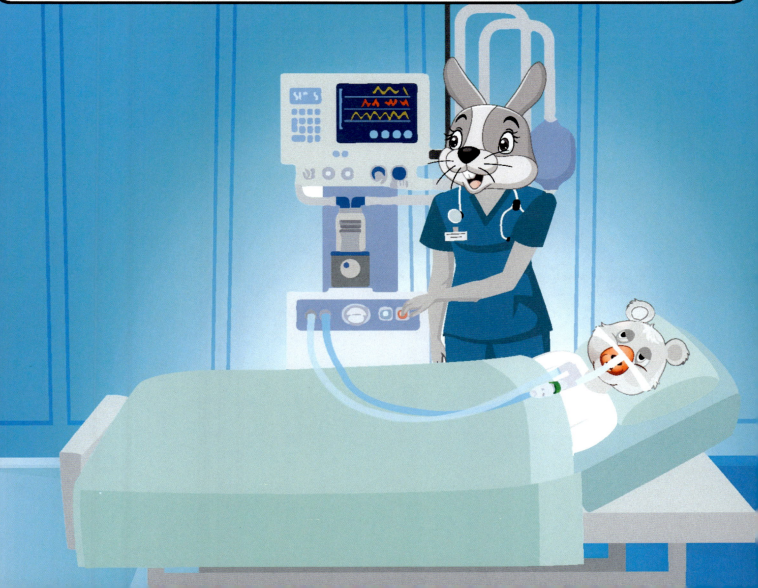

Standing at the nurse's station mom hears an alarm. She runs over to make sure there is no harm.

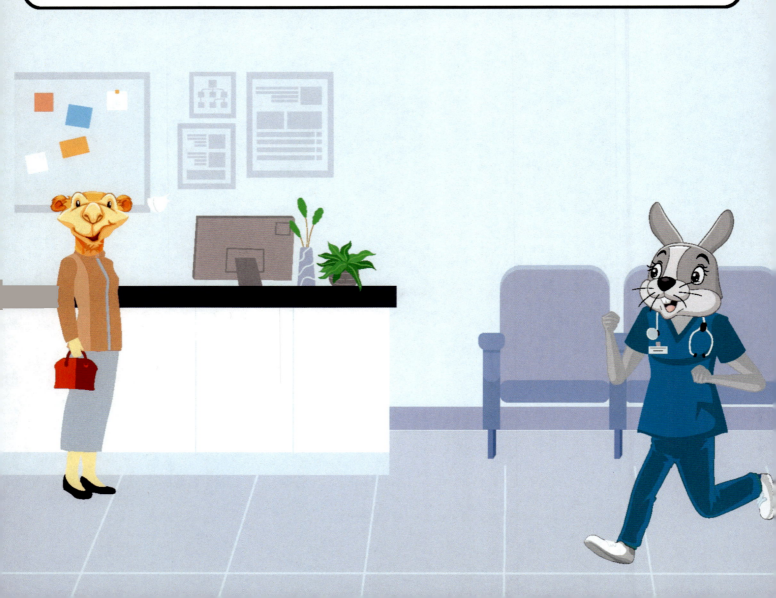

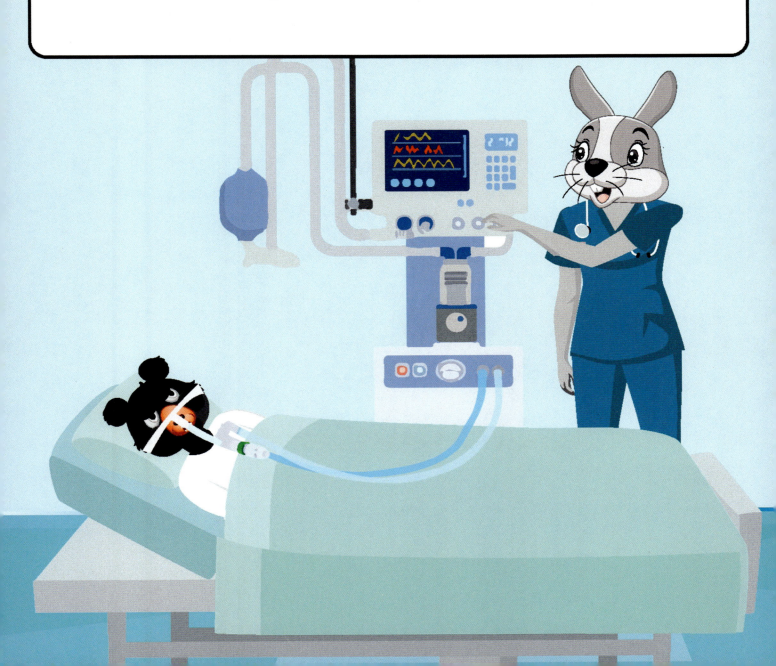

She doesn't wear a cape but sure she knows how to use ET tube tape. Keeping the patients safe and sound, so they will never frown.

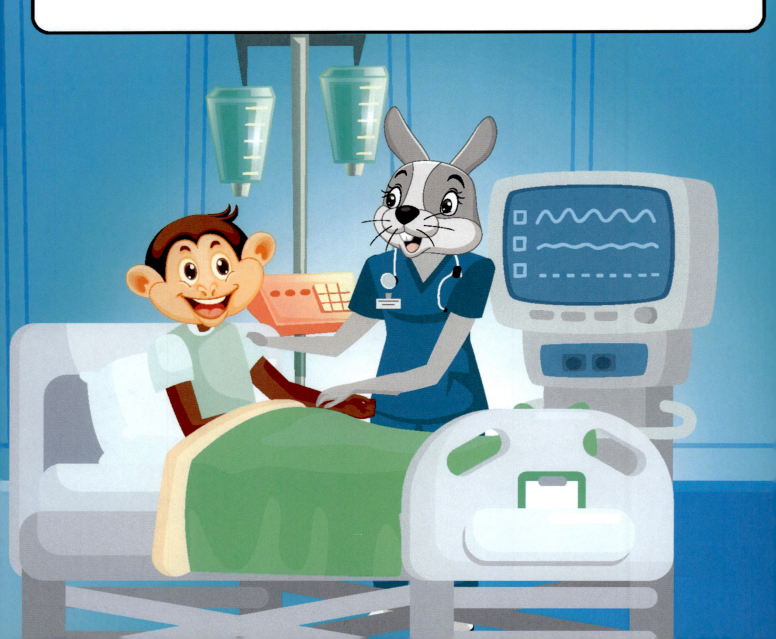

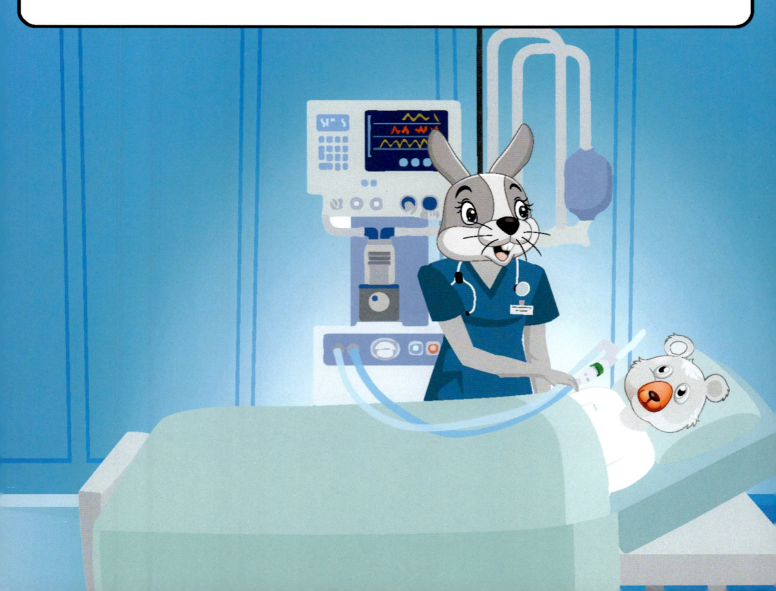

Pulling the ET tube out is the best part of her day no doubt. When the breathing tube comes out all the way, you know she had a good day.

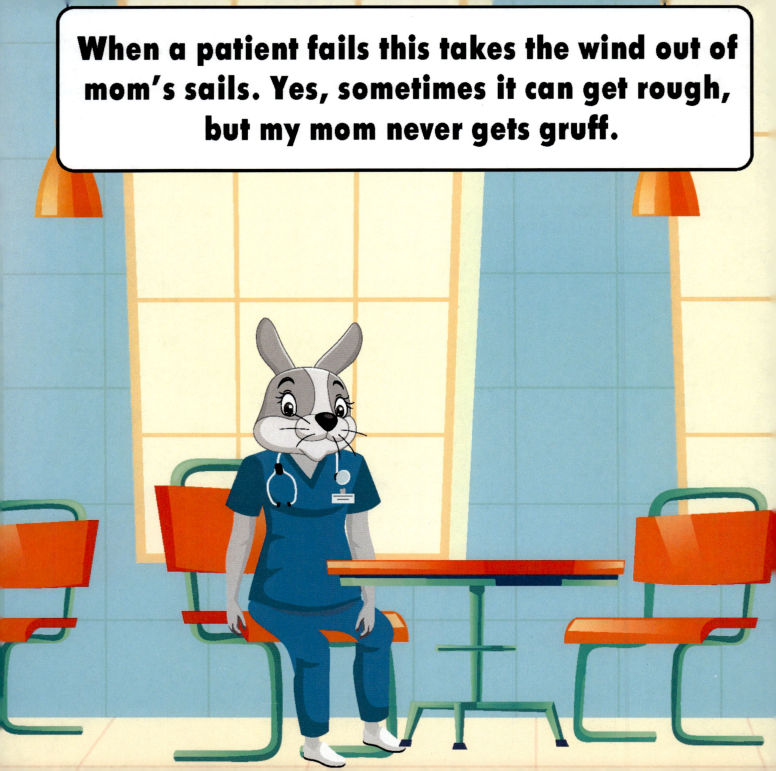

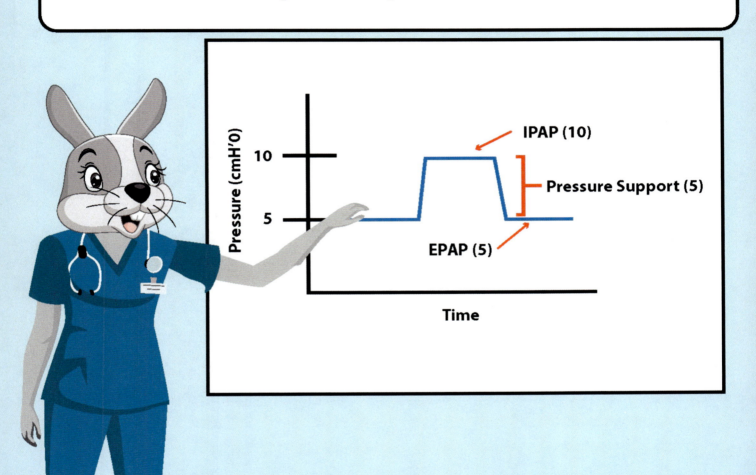

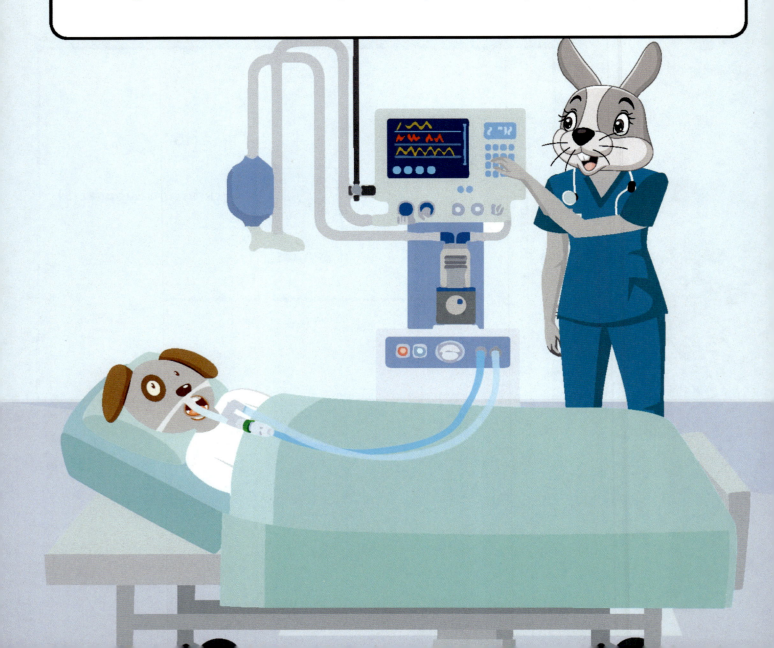

The patient gets a special glow because of all the new airflow. When this happens everyone smiles because mom knows how to turn those dials.

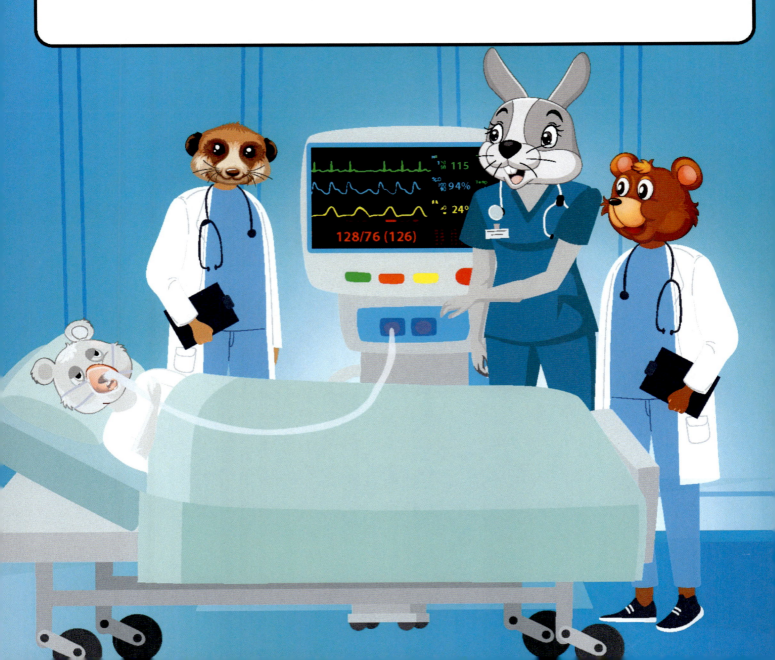

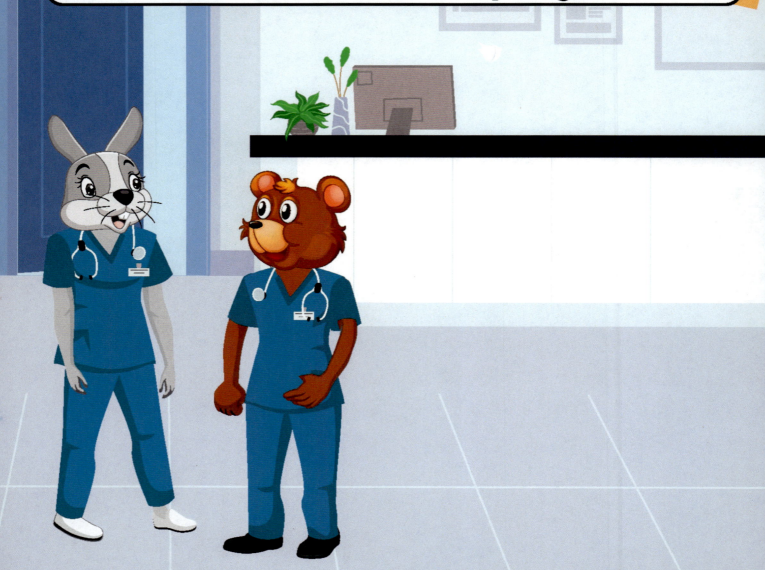

The day is finally over when mom turns around the corner. But, who does she see? Another RRT! He slept so tight. He sure does look very bright.

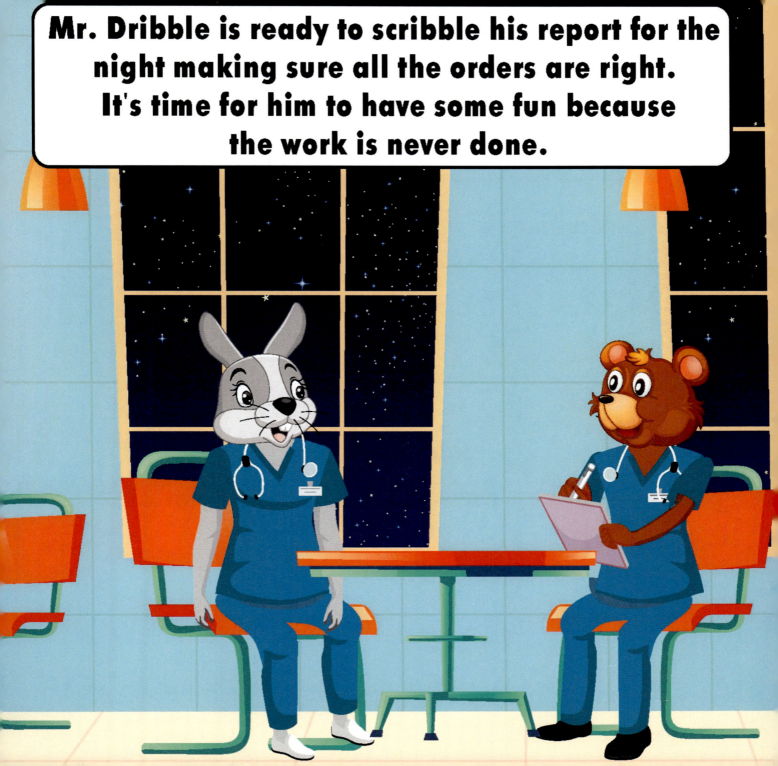

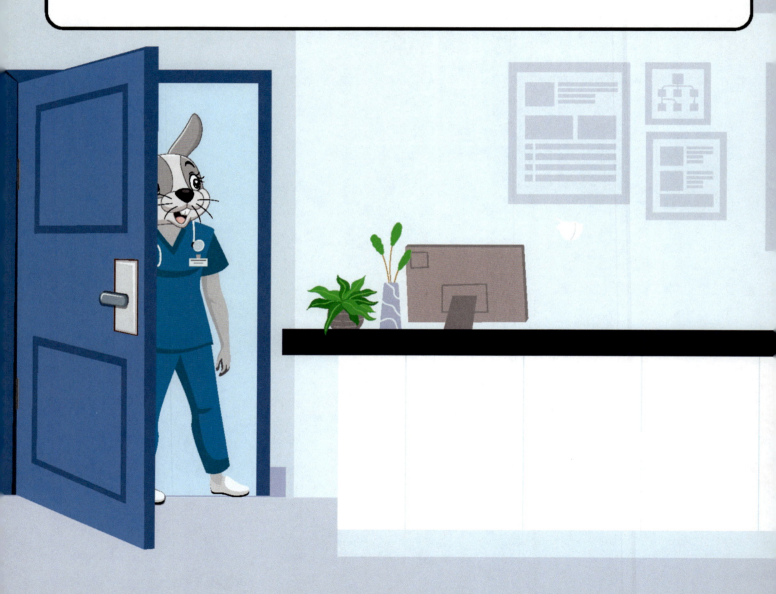

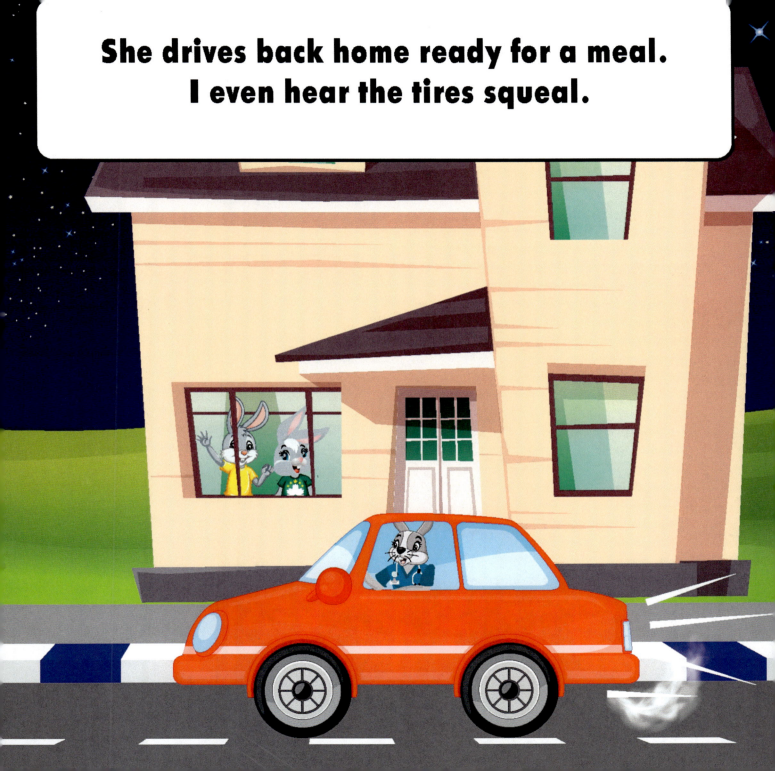

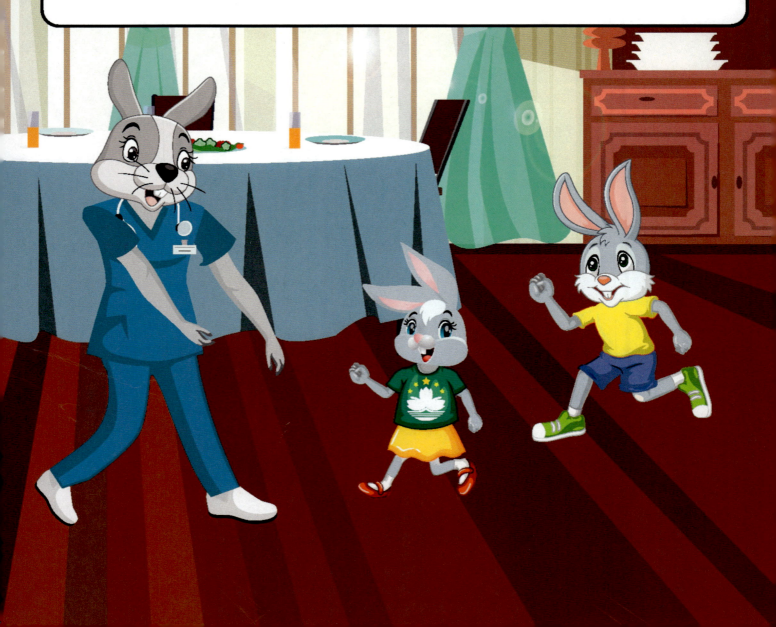

She misses and kisses us when she gets home.
It's just like when I give my dog a bone.
She is as happy as can be really just to see me.

Being an RRT is pretty cool.
It's even better than the time at the pool.

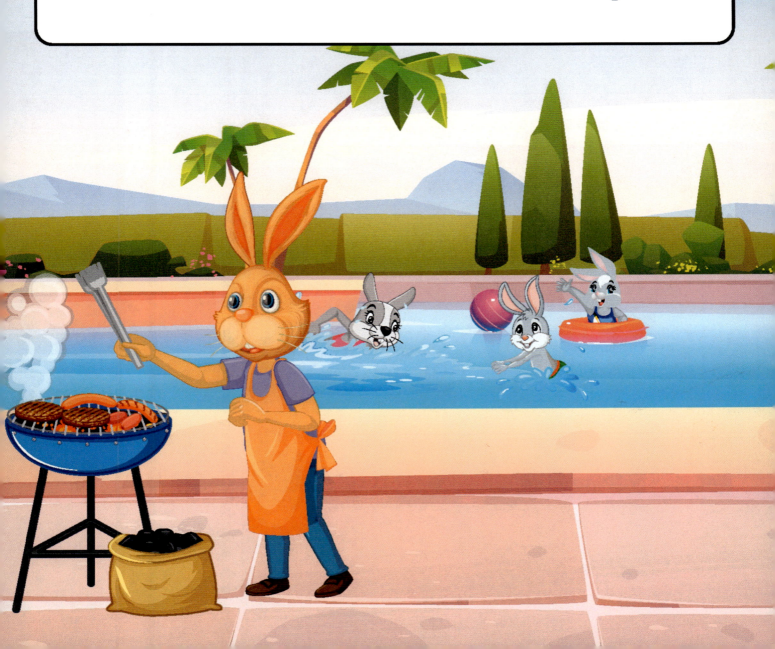

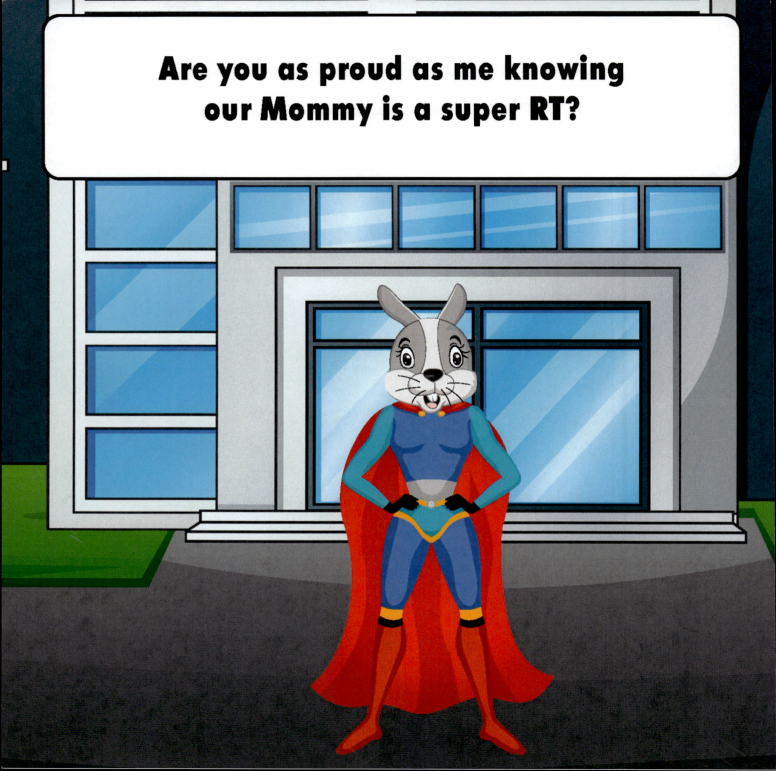

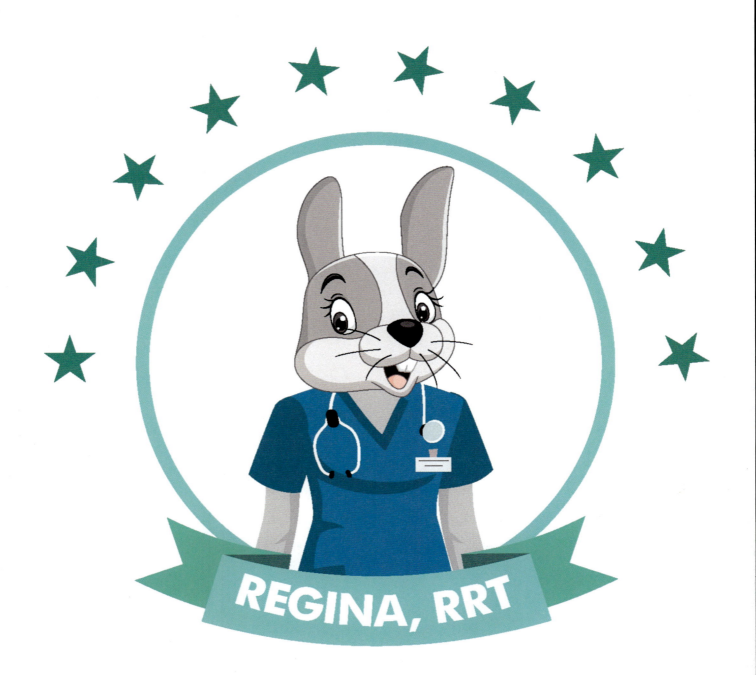

Made in the USA
Monee, IL
22 July 2021

74147171R00026